THE SHORT & TALL OF SLEEP

Increase your metabolism,
elevate your immune system
and reduce the risk of depression
and anxiety, through better sleep

Greg Justice & Art Still

Table of Contents

PART ONE

What is Sleep?

Introduction

It's arguable that there is no better feeling than lying down at night and closing your eyes. Although sleeping is often seen as lazy or a waste of time, it is actually extremely beneficial. Sliding under the covers, relaxing into a pillow, and clearing your mind of thought is perhaps the easiest way that you can help take care of your body. While working out and eating right are also very important, sleep affects the human body in countless ways that other healthy lifestyle changes can't hope to replicate. So, why do so many people neglect the importance of sleeping?

Even though it's something that everyone does every night, sleeping is still somewhat mysterious. Many people don't know what exactly happens when they close their eyes for the night. Though it may seem like sleeping just means "passing out" and then waking up in the morning, there are a dizzying number of things happening beneath the surface that affect our bodies not only at night, but also throughout the next day.

From an increased metabolism to better immunity against sicknesses and improved athletic performance to reducing the risk of depression and anxiety, the benefits of sleep are numerous. Unlike hitting the gym and physically challenging yourself in order to see results, reaping these benefits is simpler and far more pleasurable. Even so, learning to sleep better isn't going to happen overnight. Yes, that sounds counterintuitive, but it's true. Many people struggle to find adequate time to sleep thanks to busy schedules and distractions that keep us out of bed. Others struggle with problems like insomnia that make it even harder to fall asleep and stay asleep. So, while going to bed is certainly easier than sticking to a diet or workout routine, it should still be treated like those other activities. In other words, sleeping shouldn't be just another part of the day, but rather it should be treated as an important activity that deserves a priority spot in your daily routine.

Most people, when preparing to make a healthy lifestyle change, do all they can to learn about the benefits that it will have. Not only does this make someone more inclined to actually begin changing their habits, it increases the likelihood that the new changes will stick. Throughout this book, you'll learn the importance of sleep as it is framed around the many positive health benefits that come with it. Each part will focus on one aspect of sleep before breaking it down into specific examples of how sleep impacts the various systems in your body. It will also give you an easy-to-understand introduction to the science behind sleep and some common abnormalities that may affect the way you rest. Finally, you'll learn helpful tips to get more sleep and create your very own sleep goals as the first step to a healthier life. By first learning why sleeping is so important and then putting that knowledge into action, you'll be well on your way to living a more rested, healthy life.

Although sleeping is different for everybody, the importance of it cannot be understated. Uncovering the benefits of sleep is both exciting and rewarding. So, if you're ready to learn how sleep can make you healthier, then read on.

CHAPTER 1

How Much Sleep do you Really Need?

The first step towards achieving the health benefits of sleep is identifying how much sleep you actually need. Most people have heard that children and teens need more sleep than adults. While that's true to some degree, there is a significant body of research showing that the gap is far smaller than most people realize. In fact, as we progress into our older years, the need for sleep increases even more.

As such, many people don't actually know how much sleep they should be getting. Rather than basing their sleep needs off of scientifically proven data, countless people worldwide simply go based off of how they feel. If a busy parent feels "good enough" after just five hours, they are likely to stick to that schedule. If a high school student doesn't wake up tired after sleeping for six and a half hours, they might see sleeping more than that as unnecessary. However, basing a sleep schedule off of feel alone can be dangerous in the long term.

Formulating a sleep schedule based on how you feel will lead to not getting enough sleep almost every time. That's a big concern for people that are looking to harness the benefits of shut eye. A recent study showed that not getting enough sleep is actually just as harmful for your cognition as not sleeping at all. One group of participants was only allowed to sleep for six hours per night for two straight weeks. A second group slept normally but was then kept awake for two days straight prior to undergoing cognitive testing. At the end the of the research period, both groups performed equally poorly on a cognitive function test. These scary results show just how easy it is to underestimate the amount of sleep you need. To make things even worse, participants in the six hour per night group didn't even realize that they were struggling and even reported feeling just fine. Sound familiar?

Considering that approximately one-third of Americans get six hours or less per night, it's easy to see why so many people report feeling groggy and dull even though they think that they're getting enough sleep.

With these facts in mind, it is important to examine some data that suggests how much sleep we should actually be getting every night. Below, we'll examine how much sleep people should get based on their age. Notably, children under 13 aren't included in this as their sleep needs vary widely from year to year due to their complex and rapid growth and development.

Teens (Ages 13-18)

While teenagers might get a bad rap for wanting to sleep a lot, it turns out that their natural instincts aren't just being lazy. According to the Centers for Disease Control (CDC), teenagers that fall into this age group should be getting between 8-10 hours of sleep per night. Unfortunately, this need for a high number of sleeping hours coincides with the time in a teen's life when things are starting to get busy. School and homework are becoming more difficult and time-consuming, sports become more competitive, and teens are challenged to try and maintain a vibrant social life. On top of that, they are just learning stress and time management skills and don't have those abilities mastered. Combined with physiologic processes already occurring in the teenage body, getting the recommended 8-10 hours of sleep is difficult. However, it can be possible.

During adolescence, the body's natural sleep clock starts to favor a later bedtime. Research shows that most teens don't start to feel tired or ready to fall asleep until around 11:00 PM. Though many believe that teens staying up late is the root of their sleep deprivation, it's actually perfectly natural. In an ideal world, it would also be perfectly healthy. However, real life gets in the way. Considering that most middle and high schools start somewhere around 7:30 or 8:00 AM, it's easy to see how getting even the minimum of eight hours can be a challenge—let alone striving for ten.

On top of this, many teens tend to have a variable sleep schedule. In other words, they go to bed later and sleep in later on the weekends than they do throughout the week. This is perhaps the single most destructive habit that stands in the way of forming a sufficient sleep schedule. That goes for both teens and adults. As such, teens should work to maintain a consistent bedtime and wake-up time and stick to it even on the weekends.

While it might not seem fun to make sleep a priority during your teenage years, getting the recommended 8-10 hours has tremendous benefits. Waking up feeling refreshed will make getting through a long school day easier and improve extracurricular athletic performance in the afternoons. Teens who get enough sleep often perform much better in school than their peers who don't and even have a lower likelihood of developing conditions like depression and anxiety.

Adults (Ages 18-60)

For many adults, this may come as a bit of a reality check. Despite the fact that a third of adults get less than six hours of sleep per night, the CDC actually recommends getting at least seven hours or more. Undoubtedly, some people reading this are instantly thinking about how it's possible to get seven hours per night. After all, if teens thought they had it rough with school and sports, adult life gets even busier. Between work, raising kids, and the stresses that come along with being a functioning part of society, sleep is often the last thing on people's minds.

Nonetheless, sleep is just as important for adults as it is for children and teens. Since the adult body isn't developing as quickly, people between the ages of 18-60 don't need quite as much sleep as their younger counterparts. Even so, most people still don't get enough.

Sleep during the adult years is crucial to maintaining peak performance at work, in your relationships, and it plays an even bigger role in regard to your overall health. Each year that we age, our body systems slowly become more vulnerable to illness and injury. Getting enough sleep consistently allows the body to rest and heal itself. Over the long-term, this can be the difference between healthy years of retirement down the road and ones filled with doctor's appointments and prescriptions.

Older Adults (Ages 60+)

Speaking of aging, as we get leave our prime years and get older, our sleep requirements change yet again. Though many people mistakenly believe that our need for sleep decreases the older we get, adults over 60 need just as much—if not more—sleep than younger adults. The CDC recommends getting between 7-9 hours per night.

Although it seems like the retirement years would be the easiest time to get sleep since being an infant, that's not actually true. Older adults may actually struggle to fall asleep and stay asleep. During this time, sleep disturbances are often biologic and not necessarily related to environmental factors like they tend to be for younger adults. Though experts don't fully understand why this occurs, recent research points to underlying disease processes and related medications as the causes. Between the need to use the restroom in the middle of the night, insomnia, snoring, and sleep apnea, many older adults feel like they're fighting a losing battle when they lie down at night.

While there isn't a one-size-fits-all solution to falling asleep and staying asleep, falling into a regular sleep-wake rhythm can be extremely beneficial. Much like teens should try and follow a strict bedtime regimen, older adults can benefit from a similar routine.

Sleep Should Be a Priority

While the recommendations for an hourly sleep target change based on age, everyone should make getting enough sleep a priority. Whether that means sacrificing that extra episode of TV in the evening or working out during the day to make it easier to fall asleep at night, getting plenty of sleep on a consistent basis is the only way to reap the healthy benefits of it.

In today's hectic, fast-paced world, it might seem difficult to meet the sleep goals that science has proven to be the most beneficial. Inevitably, there will be nights that getting seven or eight hours simply isn't feasible. Life will get in the way. However, working to get enough sleep consistently—at least on most nights of the week—will do wonders. We'll discuss more of the benefits of sleep throughout this book. To obtain any of those, though, you need to start by getting *enough* sleep.

CHAPTER 2

Chronic Sleep Deprivation vs. Short Term Sleep Loss

Now that we've established how much sleep you should be getting; we can take a look at what happens if you don't meet that goal. It's important to note that not sleeping long enough has many more negative health effects than simply feeling tired in the morning. Moreover, the differences between chronic sleep deprivation and missing a single night of sleep are massive. Those who are chronically sleep deprived can suffer from conditions like obesity, immune system depression, caffeine dependence and more. Yet, despite the differences between the two, they often go hand in hand. Missing a single night of sleep often leads to decreased productivity the next day, more stress, and subsequently missing sleep the next night. Without some sort of control, the cycle continues to repeat itself.

With almost 70 percent of American adults not getting enough sleep on a nightly basis, both short term sleep loss and chronic sleep deprivation are growing increasingly prevalent in today's society. Everyone has felt the effects of not getting enough sleep for a night. Though chronic sleep deprivation is less common, many of us have likely fallen into it at some point—even if just temporarily. As both of these are detrimental to your health, learning about their negative effects can often be a helpful way to avoid them. By knowing how to spot the signs and symptoms of each condition, you can identify if you or a loved one is feeling the effects of a lack of sleep.

Short Term Sleep Loss

Even one night of missing or not enough sleep can start producing noticeable health effects. Consistently, this can add up and create serious problems. Think about sleep like a debt. Each day, your body is charged seven hours (the amount of sleep needed by the average adult) for the things it needs to operate. Ideally, you would repay that seven hours at the end of each day by going to bed and sleeping for that long.

Regardless of if you do or don't, though, your body is still charged an additional seven hours the next day. If you didn't repay your sleep debt, it will only continue to grow. We've already established that it is difficult for most people to get even the recommended amount of sleep—let alone trying to go above and beyond to make up for missing hours.

When you get less sleep than your body owes, you start to experience short term sleep loss. But what causes this debt in the first place? Unlike chronic sleep deprivation, which we'll discuss later, short term sleep loss is typically related to life events or emotional stress rather than a physical condition. Although not getting enough sleep for a night can be related to something like a backache or having a cold, it is more commonly caused by something other than your body. Take, for instance, a stressful day at the office. After getting yelled at by your boss and staying late to finish an important project, you'll likely find it harder to "unwind" once you get home. With work the next day looming on the horizon, you might find yourself getting to bed later than usual or having a hard time falling asleep as you dwell on the day's events. A student might experience short term sleep loss as they cram for a test into the early hours of the morning before waking up at 7:00 am. Fighting with a significant other can last into the night and cause emotional turmoil that keeps you from falling asleep. These three are just a handful of the many reasons that your nightly sleep can be disrupted.

Not surprisingly, the body doesn't like having to owe a sleep debt. It responds in turn with a host of noticeable side effects that carry on through the next day. Unlike the harmful, long-term health effects of chronic sleep loss, not getting enough Z's for one night often leads to poor performance and makes you feel like a rundown version of yourself the next day.

Short term sleep loss often creates mental issues like a lack of focus. Without an appropriate amount of sleep, your brain cannot rebalance the countless chemicals it uses to moderate everything from your mood to your energy levels. As it tries to restore order, you might find that you have difficulty focusing on important tasks and that your attention span is shortened. Oftentimes, this leads to increased stress as you struggle to accomplish your daily tasks and find them harder than usual to complete. With increased stress comes irritability and mood swings. While parents often pick up on these changes in their sleepy children, they are just as evident in adults. Missing a single night of sleep can you leave you feeling angry one minute, sad the next, and unable to control your mood swings throughout the day.

Although short term sleep loss isn't typically caused by a physical problem, it can certainly lead to them. Of course, the most noticeable side effect of not getting enough sleep is fatigue. If you are jolted awake by an alarm clock and immediately start getting ready, you might not feel it right away. However, as the day progresses, fatigue will eventually catch up. Typically, by the late afternoon (around 2:00-4:00 pm) people start to hit a rut caused by not getting enough sleep. Meanwhile, not sleeping for long enough keeps your body out of the restorative phases of deep sleep (which we will discuss in chapter three). This can leave you feeling sore and stiff in the morning since your muscles don't have enough time to relax and recover.

Most people tend to ignore the danger of not getting enough sleep for one night. However, it can be argued that the worst problem associated with short term sleep loss is that it is a slippery slope leading to chronic sleep deprivation. As their sleep debt increases with each night of not getting enough hours, a person becomes more likely to fall into bad habits. When poor sleep habits and repeated nights of less-than-optimal amounts of sleep occur, chronic sleep deprivation and its negative health problems start to set in. As such, the most important thing to remember about short-term sleep loss is that it needs to be controlled. Sometimes, it's impossible to get the recommended hours of sleep. As we've mentioned, life gets in the way. However, when that inevitably happens, you should do whatever it takes to hit your sleep target, or even exceed it, the next night. Doing so will not only help reverse the effects of short-term sleep loss, but also stave off the issues that come with its more chronic form.

Chronic Sleep Deprivation

When most people see the word chronic, they think of something that has been going on for at least several weeks but possibly even years. In the medical world, a condition is classified as chronic typically after it has been ongoing for more than six months. As such, the term chronic sleep deprivation can be misleading. Interestingly enough, chronic sleep deprivation isn't actually a true medical disorder at all. So, it can't be diagnosed on the basis of having occurred for a certain length of time. Rather, chronic sleep deprivation is the result of not getting enough sleep over "an extended period of time." This means that anyone who consistently fails to sleep for the recommended number of hours each night for anywhere from a month or more probably falls into this category. While having reoccurring sleep disturbances for multiple weeks could also probably qualify, it's likely that the underlying problem is going to keep happening and eventually fall into the same category. If it's corrected earlier, the long-term issues of chronic sleep deprivation typically disappear with it.

So, what causes a person to habitually not sleep long enough? Sometimes, the same reasons that people lose sleep in the short term can be the cause when they start forming a pattern of recurrence. However, there are many underlying conditions that can also cause chronic sleep deprivation. For example, problems that people think of as sleep disorders, such as insomnia and sleep apnea. Both of these conditions can lead to a chronic loss of sleep that continues for months, years, or even a lifetime. It's important to note that insomnia isn't the same thing as chronic sleep deprivation, but rather the first problem can lead to the latter. While insomnia is a diagnosable medical condition characterized by having trouble falling or staying asleep, chronic sleep deprivation is the result of several environmental or lifestyle factors.

While the actual cause of chronic sleep deprivation is usually diagnosed and treated by a healthcare provider, it oftentimes can't be determined until the patient recognizes that they are having symptoms. Most of these symptoms manifest themselves in one way or another, however, some can sneak by below the surface without proper screening. For example, not getting enough sleep on a consistent basis can raise a person's blood pressure over time. The compounding effect of unregulated stress hormones leads to hypertension and the many problems, such as an increased risk of heart attack and stroke, that come with it. In fact, many patients who have non-sleep related high blood pressure are told to get at least seven to eight hours of sleep as a part of their treatment plan. Meanwhile, people who develop chronic sleep deprivation can suffer from recurring headaches during the day since the brain doesn't have a chance to relax and reset. Metabolic changes associated with consistent sleep loss include a higher risk of developing obesity, type 2 diabetes, and weight gain. Finally, chronic sleep deprivation damages the body's ability to fight off infection. The immune system relies on getting enough sleep to function effectively. Not doing so on a consistent basis weakens the body's defenses and leaves you susceptible to illnesses. Chronically sleep deprived individuals often find themselves sick more often than those who get enough hours each night.

Along with these issues can come mental and social side effects as well. For instance, people who routinely wake up feeling sleep deprived are likely to turn to a cup of coffee or soda as a solution. While caffeine does help provide an energy boost for a few hours, it works in a very similar way to other drugs. Over time, your body builds up a tolerance to it. You'll eventually need more and more caffeine to get the same effect and can even start experiencing withdrawal symptoms if you go too long without it. People with caffeine dependence can have everything from a headache that won't go away to irritability to more intense fatigue than before. Meanwhile, the psychological changes related to chronic sleep deprivation might be harder to pick up on since they come on gradually. Nonetheless, people can start to experience personality changes, memory impairment, hallucinations, symptoms that mimic ADHD, and severe mood swings. Oftentimes, these changes are more easily detected by a loved one or roommate.

How to Fight Back

Reading about the many negative effects of not getting enough sleep, either on a short-term or long-term basis, can be scary. It might also feel a bit like reading your own biography if you are currently suffering from these symptoms. Fortunately, fighting back against a lack of sleep is possible with a consistent routine and some dedicated lifestyle changes.

Instead of feeling fatigued, stressed, irritable, and unhealthy, you can start reaping the benefits of sleep. Like all things, understanding that there is a problem is the first step. If you think that you are experiencing some form of sleep debt, then keep reading. The rest of this book will discuss the many positive benefits of sleep and help you identify ways to start getting enough of it. If you think that short term sleep loss and chronic sleep deprivation don't apply to you, then perhaps you really are sleeping long enough. However, there's a reason that you picked up this book in the first place. In all likelihood, you could be doing a better job of getting enough sleep. Perhaps try asking those close to you if you've displayed any of the symptoms discussed in this chapter. It might be an eye-opening experience that will motivate you to keep your eyes shut for longer at bedtime.

CHAPTER 3

Sleep Cycles

Have you ever wondered why being woken up by an alarm clock feels so different from allowing your body to wake up naturally? There's actually a scientific explanation for that. It all revolves around the different stages of sleep. If you are jolted awake from a deep, rapid eye movement (REM) sleep, you're going to feel groggier than waking up from a light sleep stage. Conversely, scheduling a power nap designed to wake you up from the second stage of non-REM sleep can leave you feeling refreshed and energized. Though it's extremely difficult to track sleep stages at home, understanding how they work in a general sense can make getting enough sleep easier.

This chapter will break down the several stages of sleep. It will also outline the health benefits that are associated with each stage. Believe it or not, REM sleep provides far different benefits than light, non-REM sleep. While all of the stages are important, seeing how each of them plays a part in the overall sleep routine is both fascinating and eye-opening.

Non-REM Versus REM Sleep

At its most basic, sleep can be divided into two levels: REM and non-REM. When you first fall asleep, your body enters a state of non-REM rest that is very light. Each stage is divided based on how much brain activity is occurring and how your body reacts. Furthermore, the different stages of sleep vary in length from about seven minutes in the shortest one to lengthy 30-60-minute REM cycles.

In essence, non-REM sleep is a progressive pathway that brings you from the semi-conscious state you'd feel while taking a five-minute "catnap" to the dream-filled waves of REM. Non-REM is further broken down into three distinct stages. Stage N1 is the lightest sleep while stage N3 is the deepest. We'll move through the sleep stages in the same order that your body does.

Stage N1: Transition Sleep

When you close your eyes and start to "drift away" your body enters stage N1 sleep. Within minutes, eye movements begin to slow down and the brain starts to emit alpha and theta waves. While these are detectable to a brain monitor, you won't notice any changes. In fact, people in N1 sleep can be easily awoken by very light stimuli. Saying someone's name, a loud noise, or even a sudden change in temperature can pull a person out of this stage.

Often, stage N1 is described as the change period from being awake to being asleep. However, since the body is naturally good at falling asleep, this stage is brief. In most cases, stage N1 only lasts about seven minutes—though it can extend to around 10 minutes.

Throughout stage N1, the body begins to prepare itself for sleep. Your heart rate and breathing slow down and your muscles begin to relax. Some people notice occasional twitching during this phase. While twitching can happen for everyone, it's widely believed that males twitch more than females in stage N1.

If a person isn't interrupted in this phase, they'll seamlessly transition into stage N2.

Stage N2: Light Sleep

In essence, stage N2 sleep is just a continued version of N1. During this time, the brain, heart, breathing, and muscles relax even further. In addition, body temperature begins to fall. People in this stage display brief spikes in brain activity known as sleep spindles. In general, however, brain waves continue to slow down during stage N2.

Often referred to simply as "light sleep," stage N2 is the most common among all repeated sleep phases and people fall into it more than all other stages of REM and non-REM. Like N1, stage N2 sleep doesn't come with many health benefits of its own. Instead, it serves as a starting point for sleep cycles that's even closer to the more restful stages of N3 and REM. Unfortunately, people who are highly stressed, have poor sleep habits, and those who are older spend more time sleeping lightly. This means that they are deprived of the benefits of deeper sleep.

Nonetheless, stage N2 can be beneficial for those taking a nap throughout the day. It is a perfect mid-range sleep for people catching approximately 30 minutes of shut eye perhaps on a lunch break or after school. Light sleep allows the brain to rest but waking up from it is still easy. This combination can leave a person feeling refreshed with an extra burst of energy to finish out the day. Comparatively, sharply waking up from a deeper sleep stage can leave you feeling even more tired.

In terms of sleeping at night, however, stage N2 will come and go many times. From it, our body can progress into the deep healing sleep of stage N3 and the memory-boosting sleep of REM.

Stage N3: Deep Sleep

The transition between stages N2 and N3 is significant. This occurs during the first half of the night in long periods. In stage N3, the body slows down a great deal and your heart rate and breathing drop to their lowest levels. Your muscles relax fully and your eyes also still. As the brain starts to produce large amounts of delta waves, the body becomes highly unresponsive to external stimuli. Appropriately, this stage is simultaneously known as delta sleep. From here, it's very difficult to rouse someone.

Of all of the four phases of sleep, N3 is arguably the most important. Since the body is totally relaxed, it takes this time to regenerate tissues and bones thanks to an increased release of growth hormone. Stage N3 also helps strengthen the immune system against attack. Finally, the deep relaxation state allows your brain and body to recover. Those who get enough deep sleep will wake up in the morning feeling refreshed and energized.

From stage N3, sleepers progress to the final phase: REM.

REM Sleep

While the progression of stages N1-N3 see the body relax more with each transition, REM takes things in the opposite direction. About 90 minutes after first falling asleep, brain waves start to resemble what they look like when a person is awake. Along with this, your eyes start to move rapidly behind your closed eyelids. Your heart rate and blood pressure also increase until they are near your wakefulness levels. Strangely enough, your limbs actually become paralyzed temporarily in this stage. Those who are suddenly woken up from REM sleep may feel this effect for several seconds or minutes as their body tries to catch up.

However, what most people know REM sleep for is the dreams that occur during it. Though some may experience occasional dreaming in other stages, it almost always happens during REM. As REM sleep is more common in the second half of the night, many people wake up slowly from a dream and can remember it in the morning.

Meanwhile, REM sleep plays an important role in memory and cognition. During this time, the brain consolidates and sorts through the vast quantities of information that we experience throughout the day. Some believe that dreaming is the result of this process. Regardless, getting enough REM sleep is crucial for enhancing memories of past events as much of a person's long-term memory is developed while they are in this stage.

Repeat Cycles

With a better understanding of the various sleep stages, it should become easier to see how not getting enough sleep can lead to negative side effects. For instance, not getting enough hours in bed can lead to a decrease in REM sleep and a poorer ability to recall information the next day. Likewise, going to bed with a high stress level can lead to less stage N3 deep sleep that leaves you feeling unenergized in the morning.

As we sleep, our body repeatedly cycles through these stages. Generally, you go through each one about five or six times.

With this information in mind, we'll dive deeper into the physical benefits of sleep as a whole in part two.

Physical Benefits of Sleep

CHAPTER 4

How Sleep Affects Your Immune System

As we dive into the physical health benefits of sleep, it makes sense to start with the body system that is perhaps singlehandedly responsible for keeping us healthy: the immune system. The amount of sleep a person gets each night heavily influences how effective the immune system is and whether it is able to perform its daily disease-fighting functions. Humans rely on a complex chain of antibodies, memory cells, and attack cells to stave off invading pathogens. Though research is still conflicting about how exactly sleep affects these mechanisms, it has conclusively shown that getting enough hours of sleep nightly does indeed bolster the immune system's defenses.

It's important to note that not getting enough sleep isn't actually going to make you sick. After all, just because you didn't go to bed doesn't mean you've been exposed to a virus or bacteria. By contrast, we are constantly being exposed to tens of thousands of strains and species of pathogens every day. A lack of sleep hinders your immune system from fighting off invaders that you do come in contact with. Long-term sleep deprivation will compound these issues, putting the immune system at an even steeper disadvantage.

Sleeping prepares your immune system for its strenuous tasks in two different ways. First, it allows for the production of cytokines, a type of protein that decreases inflammation. In addition to this, the low-energy, relaxed state of sleep allows immune cells to "recharge" for the next day and prepare to mount a response to infection.

Sleep Bolsters Cytokine Production

The concept of cytokines can be a difficult one for those not familiar with the medical field. In essence, cytokines are a collection of different proteins that either promote or antagonize inflammation by carrying signals between cells in the body. Of course, when most people think of the word "inflammation," it automatically gets a negative connotation. Contrary to popular belief, some inflammation is actually a necessary part of the immune system's disease fighting process. While some cytokines promote inflammation, such as those that respond to an injury, the ones produced during sleep mainly help inhibit high levels of inflammation. The mechanisms in which cytokines regulate the immune system are extremely complex. As such, we won't dive into the detailed science behind how they work. However, on a basic level, they primarily activate immune system cells and also direct them to where they are needed in the body. For example, if you cut your arm, cytokines will tell white blood cells to rush to the area and devour any invading pathogens.

Studies show that the body both produces and releases a wide variety of cytokines during sleep. Accordingly, not getting enough of it can lead to decreased cytokine availability, thus weakening the immune system. Without cytokines to guide disease-fighting processes, the body is more likely to succumb to an illness. In times when pathogens are more prevalent than usual, like during flu season, not getting enough sleep can almost guarantee a bout of sickness.

Since cytokines direct the immune system's memory mechanisms as well, not getting enough sleep can also decrease the effectiveness of vaccines. To use flu season as an example again, a person who is experiencing chronic sleep deprivation when they get their flu shot won't be able to properly build up an immunity like someone that is well rested.

Finally, the anti-inflammatory cytokines produced during sleep help prevent complications from having too much inflammation. Over time, people who don't get enough sleep are put at a higher risk for problems like autoimmune diseases that occur when the body's inflammatory processes spiral out of control. Sleeping helps maintain an ideal balance of having healthy, disease-fighting inflammation and not having too much of it.

Your Immune System Needs Rest, Too

Later on, we'll discuss how sleep gives the body's vital organs a chance to rest and recover from their taxing daily routines. Although the immune system is primarily made up of cells and not large organs (excluding the spleen) it also needs to rest. Sleeping allows it to do just that. As the body settles into the latter stages of deep sleep, immune system cells move out of the normal circulation and into specialized bundles of tissue known as lymph nodes. Lymph is a fluid that flows throughout its own network in the body and collects waste products. The specialized nodes filter these substances out before returning the clean fluid to the bloodstream. Inside the lymph nodes, immune system cells have a chance to "recharge" and prepare for the coming day. While resting, these intelligent cells are exposed to foreign antigens and are able to begin the process of adaptive immunity. Ultimately, this allows them to detect and destroy invading pathogens before they can create a systemic illness. Without sleep, or with less of it, immune system cells don't receive the same exposure to these antigens and can't begin mounting a response as quickly or effectively.

Although the brain isn't maintained by the lymphatic network, it has a similar process for cleaning out toxic wastes and inflammation. During sleep, these substances are removed, which leads to healthier tissue and better function upon waking.

Add Vitamin Sleep

While sleeping has tremendous physiologic effects on the immune system, it is still only one part of the immunity equation. Simply getting the recommended number of hours of sleep each night isn't a miracle way to keep yourself free of disease. If it were, perhaps more people would make sleeping a priority. Nonetheless, being well-rested is an important part of maintaining a healthy immune system. When combined with other interventions, it can make a significant difference in a person's general state of wellness.

Along with getting enough sleep, everyone should take some basic measures to aid their immune system in its constant battle. For one, proper hand hygiene makes a huge difference. Tri-County Health Care suggests that there are an estimated 2-10 million individual bacteria living between your fingertips and elbows at any given time. Meanwhile, approximately 80 percent of illness-causing germs are spread your hands. These figures show why handwashing is so important. The CDC claims that 1 in 3 diarrhea-related sicknesses and 1 in 5 respiratory illnesses can be prevented by handwashing alone. By combining proper hand hygiene with a well-balanced diet and a schedule with plenty of sleep, you can give your body the best possible chance of avoiding illness.

The immune system is truly an awe-inspiring, coordinated defense mechanism. However, if it is deprived of the tools that it needs to succeed, it will eventually fail. By doing something as simple as sleeping for the recommended number of hours each night, you automatically help strengthen it against all natures of foreign invaders.

CHAPTER 5

Sleep and Your Cardiovascular Health

Heart health is one of the biggest topics discussed in the medical world today. From cereal that promises to decrease your risk of heart disease to supplements designed to keep your heart healthy, everyone focuses on this vital organ. Considering that the cardiovascular system is the body's way of supplying materials essential for life in the form of oxygen and nutrients, there's a good reason for society's concern with it. While people know that exercise and eating a low-fat diet is good for heart health, not everyone is familiar with the fact that sleep plays an important role in supporting the circulatory system as well. Perhaps that is because scientists still aren't sure exactly how sleep affects the heart and blood vessels. Nonetheless, countless studies have shown that a positive correlation exists between getting enough sleep and having better heart health. Meanwhile, blood pressure is known to decrease during sleep, which gives the body a chance to recover from the high levels that may occur during the day.

It shouldn't be a surprise that sleeping more can lead to better heart health. While getting some Z's does great things for the cardiovascular system, it can only happen if you're getting enough sleep. As discussed in previous chapters, adult should be getting—at a minimum—7 hours each night. By hitting this target consistently, the benefits of sleep will start to take effect. Prior to jumping into the specifics of how sleeping more can benefit your heart, let's look at an overview of what the cardiovascular system is and what it does.

What is the Cardiovascular System?

While many people think of the cardiovascular system only as the heart, it is far more than that. It is a complex network of arteries and veins that transport blood throughout the body at a rate that matches its ever-changing demand. Along with the nervous system and respiratory system, it is one of the most important processes that sustains life.

Each day, the heart pumps more than 100,000 times. That adds up to more than 42 million beats per year. It never stops and never gets a chance to rest. As such, this amazing muscle deserves some extra attention. The heart must overcome several obstacles in its effort to pump blood around the body. One of the most important ones is blood pressure. While adequate pressure is needed to provide blood to organs like the kidneys, pressure that is too high can be detrimental. The higher the blood pressure is, the harder the heart must work to push blood into the systemic circulation. People who have high blood pressure are subsequently at a higher risk for other cardiovascular problems like having a stroke or heart attack.

Meanwhile, high blood pressure can directly damage organs and tissues in the body. Many diabetics also suffer from high blood pressure and eventually develop vision problems as a result. When the pressure is too high over a long period of time, it can cause damage to the small vessels throughout the body. These detrimental issues are known as microvascular complications. However, high blood pressure doesn't just affect small vessels. It can also lead to poor oxygenation in the kidneys and even the heart itself. High blood pressure causes these macrovascular complications when it affects larger organs.

Since high blood pressure increases the risk of both types of complications, maintaining a healthy level should be a priority for everyone. Though a doctor's recommendations may vary, the normal level for a blood pressure is 120/80 mmHg. Activities like aerobic exercise, low-fat diets, and, of course, getting enough sleep are all tools to help manage blood pressure. Those who struggle to keep their numbers low may also need to take medications. However, the most natural option is always the best first resort. In this case, sleeping for at least 7 hours per night is the easiest contribution towards a lower blood pressure and a healthier cardiovascular system.

Sleep Lowers the Heart Rate and Blood Pressure

Chapter 3 discussed the various stages of sleep that the body progresses through each night. The longer we stay asleep, the more time we spend in the latter, deeper stages. In these periods of relaxation, the heart rate actually slows down as the body's demand for energy and blood flow decreases. Although a heart rate that is too slow can be a bad thing, the American Heart Association says that it may often fall below 60 beats per minute during sleep. Not only is this normal, it's healthy. This slower pace gives the heart a chance to rest before increasing its rhythm and workload to meet the demands of the day.

Sleep doesn't only lower the heart rate though. For the same reasons outlined above, blood vessels also relax during sleep. As they relax, the blood pressure decreases. While experts aren't quite sure why this change occurs, several studies have confirmed that it is a common event. Some have even shown that systolic blood pressure can drop by as much as 15 mmHg from daytime levels when a person is sleeping. This change doesn't just affect the body at night, however. It can also influence blood pressure levels over the course of time by "training" the body to relax its vessels.

Sleep Apnea and Blood Pressure

While most people that sleep through the night are able to harness the benefits of lower blood pressure, some are not. For instance, those with sleep apnea. People suffering from this disorder are repeatedly woken up at night when their breathing spontaneously stops. While sleep apnea can be caused by other conditions, primarily obesity, it can lead to negative cardiovascular effects as well. Experts have identified a strong link between sleep apnea and the development of heart problems. One study found that men with severe sleep apnea are 58 percent more likely to develop congestive heart failure later in life than those without the sleep disorder. It is believed that an increase in excitatory chemicals is to blame for this correlation.

Better Sleep Decreases the Risk of Heart Disease

For everyone, not just those who have sleep apnea, getting enough sleep at night is crucial to maintaining good heart health. Just like the immune system, sleep alone won't maintain a healthy heart. A combination of a good diet, daily exercise, and controlled weight works together to make the entire cardiovascular system function better and more effectively. Nonetheless, getting enough sleep benefits the heart and many other systems at the same time. To help achieve the best cardiovascular health, be sure to get the recommended 7 hours of sleep each night. Your heart will thank you for it and you'll be at a lower risk of developing cardiovascular-related problems as you age.

CHAPTER 6

Sleep Improves Athletic Performance

Although a good hard practice can make anyone ready to put their head on a pillow for the night, not all athletes think about their sleep. Even fewer think about how it affects their athletic performance. Of course, not getting enough sleep can leave a player feeling groggy and sluggish when they take the field (or court, or any other sports setting). On the flipside, taking a nap too close to game time can leave a player's muscles feeling stiff and tired. However, new research is beginning to show that getting the recommended amount of sleep or more can actually boost athletic performance. A large part of this has to do with the body's natural recovery process. For athletes, this is even more important than it is for an everyday person.

At the same time, no matter the sport, all athletes require two things to function at their best: quick cognitive function and long-lasting endurance. During rigorous exercise and hours of practice, muscle tissue is damaged and nutrients are depleted. Getting enough sleep helps restore these things and many more. On top of this, increased sleep helps improve focus at game time and can lead to better performance in the heat of the moment. As such, achieving the optimal length of sleep each night can give athletes an advantage over the competition.

Sleep Leads to Better Athletic Performance

When it comes to finding ways to enhance their performance, athletes have all sorts of superstitious rituals. From throwing chalk in the air to wearing a certain jacket to the field, most players are willing to do whatever it takes to perform at their best. So, why don't more athletes focus on getting enough sleep the night before a game?

Studies show that sleeping more is associated with enhanced accuracy and reaction times, less fatigue, and even more anaerobic power. Of course, regardless of what sport an athlete participates in, these things are highly important. Without the need for lucky socks, more sleep can lead to better athletic performance and should be an important part of every player's pre-game (and everyday) ritual.

Plenty of sports rely on pinpoint accuracy for success. Games like basketball, soccer, and hockey require athletes to focus on a relatively small spot and get the ball or puck there as fast as possible. A study of collegiate male basketball players found that those who increased their nightly sleep by two hours over a five to seven-week period saw nine percent increases in both free throw and three-point field goal accuracy. Likewise, a 1.6 hour increase in sleep time helped collegiate tennis players achieve 36% to 41% more accurate serves. These studies, among many others, show that increasing one's amount of sleep on a consistent basis can lead to increased accuracy across a variety of sports.

Athletes in every sport can benefit from less fatigue. After all, it's impossible to perform at your peak when you're feeling worn down. While this may be the most obvious benefit of getting more sleep, it is still often overlooked. Yet, athletes who sleep more experience less fatigue during their sporting events. That shouldn't be a surprising fact. Getting more sleep also helps athletes up their mental game. When it comes down to crunch time and outlasting an opponent is the key to victory, being able to put fatigue aside and continue performing is a game-winning trait. It's one that is seen in professional athletes across the sports spectrum and one that coaches value tremendously. Unfortunately, studies have shown that there is less glycogen stored in the muscles prior to exercise in people who are sleep deprived. This means that athletes working on less sleep also have less fuel as the game goes on. Meanwhile, endurance tests in the lab have shown that athletes who sleep more have a lower rating of perceived exertion than those who are lacking sleep. As such, getting more sleep seems to directly influence how tired an athlete actually thinks they are. In a make or break moment, knowing that you have more to give can be all a player needs to keep going. On the flipside, sleep deprived players will have to fight against their brain, which is telling them that they're exhausted, to maintain their energy level. It's obvious to see which athlete has the edge at the end of a game.

Not every game depends on anaerobic muscle power in the same way. However, sports like football, wrestling, and baseball rely on how much strength an athlete is able to generate during bursts of anaerobic muscle activity. Current research is still split regarding the effect of sleep on this type of performance. While it appears that not getting enough sleep in a single night affects anaerobic strength less than it does endurance, consecutive nights of sleep deprivation do lead to poorer results in various tests. Athletes put through Wingate testing (a stationary bike trial designed to test leg muscle strength) had significantly decreased power outputs after being sleep deprived for 36 hours. Similarly, a study of young adult males found that maximal weight lifts decreased after getting three consecutive nights with three hours of sleep or less. So, although not getting enough sleep doesn't affect anaerobic muscle performance as readily as endurance performance, it is still worth noting. Getting enough sleep consistently can help athletes achieve their peak levels of strength.

How Sleep Affects Athletic Recovery

Although sleep's effect on athletic performance while on the playing field is massive, the role it plays in recovery after exercise cannot be understated. Regardless of the sport being played or the workout being performed, exercise depletes the body of many things. Primarily, it leaves athletes in a deficit of both fluids and energy. Likewise, exercise breaks down muscle. While this process is necessary for rebuilding the muscles to make them stronger, it can't be completed without adequate recovery. Although proper hydration and eating are major parts of that recovery, sleep shouldn't be overlooked either. The body uses the relaxed state of sleep as an opportunity to release many of its hormones. One of these is human growth hormone (HGH). Though HGH gets a bad rap as something athletes illegally take as a supplement to enhance their performance, it's actually a natural part of the body's self-healing process. The hormone contributes to the repair of muscles and other tissues that are damaged during athletic participation. There's a reason that some professional athletes try to get extra of it. HGH is one of the most important substances for helping the body heal and get stronger.

Fortunately, athletes don't have to turn to illegal supplements to boost their levels of HGH and, subsequently, their recovery. The stages of deep sleep that occur when a person increases their amount of time in bed also happen to be the peak times for HGH release. Most experts agree that about 75 percent of HGH is released during sleep. For athletes who skimp out on a nightly routine, this means that their recovery process is at a severe disadvantage. By contrast, those who get seven to nine hours of sleep per night on a regular basis can heal and recover faster and more effectively than their non-sleeping opponents.

Sleep Wins Championships

Interestingly enough, there have been several studies done to correlate how getting more sleep affects athletic performance. Most of these take place in the NCAA setting as college student-athletes are more apt to participate in a study than professional players. However, the results apply to athletes of all ages. One researcher from Stanford is quoted as saying, "If people understood how much of a difference getting more sleep could make athletically, they'd incorporate it into their lives and not focus solely on nutrition and exercise." It's that line of thinking that goes to show how important sleep is in relation to athletic performance. However, the results of several studies from Stanford also speak for themselves.

Elite NCAA athletes from Stanford University's swim team (men's and women's) took place in a study to measure how their sleep levels affected their performance in meets. During the first two weeks of the study, the swimmers maintained their normal sleep schedule. For the next two weeks, they proceeded to increase their sleep to 10 hours per night. Researchers measured the performance of the athletes in both phases of the study. The results are incredible. After getting more sleep, athletes saw faster lap times, quicker reaction times from the starting blocks, and even faster turn times. Some of the swimmers also went on to set school and NCAA records during the course of the study. Meanwhile, a similar study of the school's women's basketball team found that every player on the team made more shots and ran faster when they got 10 hours of sleep per night. Interestingly enough, that same team went on to compete for the NCAA Championship that year.

While these are simply the results of one study, they do an excellent job of illustrating the impact that sleep can have on athletic performance. There are even more studies that have come to similar conclusions with their own results. All of this goes to say, getting more sleep might just be the advantage that a team or a player needs to reach the pinnacle of their game and win a championship.

Sleep Good, Play Good

Athletes are willing to push their body to the limit in order to get better at their sport. Whether that means showing up early and staying late after practice or pushing past exhaustion in the fourth quarter, competitors do whatever it takes to get better and get the win. For any athlete, getting enough sleep is the easiest way to help ensure that your performance is at its peak and that your body can recover. Without it, the endless hours of practice and weight room workouts are meaningless. However, by following sleep guidelines and getting enough hours each night, athletes will see improvements in their game both physically and mentally.

CHAPTER 7

Sleeping Well Regulates Your Metabolism

No one would complain about having a faster metabolism. Most people can remember the increased metabolism of their youth. Being able to eat anything without gaining weight back then didn't seem like the luxury it is in adulthood. According to the 2013-14 National Health and Nutrition Examination Survey, more than two thirds of American adults are either overweight or obese. Likewise, approximately one in six children under the age of 19 in the United States are considered obese. Since that survey is now a few years old, it's likely that the percentages are even higher. While a large portion of America's weight problem is due to the poor dietary habits and food choices in the country, lifestyle factors also play a role in the way that the body processes food and uses energy. Studies have shown that sleep deprivation can lead to a slower metabolism that can cause weight gain over time if left untreated. On the flip side, getting enough sleep every night can help keep the body's metabolism running at its best. A strong metabolism can even lead to mild weight loss and better overall health.

The Vicious Sleep Deprivation Cycle

Unfortunately, sleep deprivation doesn't just lead to fatigue. Nor does it only lead to weight gain. Instead, it causes a vicious cycle of side-effects that all contribute to and make each other worse. The longer this goes on, the more likely it is to lead to serious complications like developing diabetes or having a BMI that climbs into the range of obese to morbidly obese. While it's hard to isolate the symptoms from each other, there is one bright side. Altering one's sleep schedule to include the recommended seven or more hours each night can actually stop the cycle in its tracks. Despite the fact that sleep deprivation can lead to an array of side effects from hormonal imbalances to a dip in energy levels, increasing the amount of time spent sleeping can alleviate all of them. Not often does one lifestyle change make such a big difference.

So, where exactly does this cycle start? It's no surprise that it begins with fatigue. After all, that is the most direct side-effect of not getting enough sleep. Those with a busy schedule or who simply don't prioritize sleep will wake up feeling groggy, tired, and unmotivated. As this trend continues over a period of time, the fatigue only gets worse. Studies have shown that, during sleep, the body produces more of a hormone known as leptin and less of one called ghrelin. The latter is the body's signal that it is hungry. It leads to the grumbling stomach and cravings that a person experiences when they haven't eaten in a long time. By contrast, leptin comes from fat tissue and tells the body that it has enough resources and acts as an antagonist to ghrelin. Studies have shown that the body produces more leptin while it is asleep. This helps prevent you from waking up due to hunger cues. One of these studies, which restricted participants to two hours of sleep per night, found that leptin levels were decreased by as much as 18 percent at the end of the trial. Ultimately, this led participants to crave sweet, starchy, and salty foods more than they did normally. Of course, these descriptors don't match many healthy foods.

This highlights the second step in the cycle of sleep deprivation. The combination of fatigue and decreased leptin levels often leads people to eat poorly during the day. When a person feels lethargic, they might reach for something like a candy bar or a donut as a quick pick-me-up. Cravings related to lower leptin levels may also encourage someone to eat more fast food or processed foods that are high in fat and sodium. This is an example of what scientists call "nonhomeostatic food intake." In essence, it is when a person is consuming food for emotional or psychological reasons (such as in response to a craving) and not because the body needs the calories. Most of the time when this occurs, those extra calories simply end up getting turned into adipose tissue and stored as fat. Moreover, these unhealthy foods don't provide long-term energy for those who are already tired. So, a person is left feeling worn out but now has a weight gain problem to deal with as well.

Less Sleep = Less Exercise

The sleep deprivation cycle doesn't only affect eating choices. Rather, the fatigue associated with chronic sleep loss also leads to further negative health behaviors. When considering weight gain or loss, exercising is always a part of the discussion. In fact, exercise has been shown to be one of the best ways to help lose weight—along with eating a balanced, portioned diet. However, no one is ready to go on a run or hit the weights when they wake up in the morning feeling tired and sore already.

The fatigue associated with chronic sleep loss only compounds over time as the sleep debt grows. While exercise can help boost energy levels, it is extremely difficult to make it a habit when even a moderately intense workout leaves you feeling exhausted. Those getting less than seven hours of sleep per night often want nothing to do with the gym and are simply trying to get through the day without falling asleep at their desk. Unfortunately, even those who are able to push past the fatigue and get a workout in won't reap all of the benefits of it. As discussed in the previous chapter, those who don't get enough sleep experience an inhibited recovery following athletic performance. They also have less endurance and cannot perform as well as someone who has gotten more sleep.

On the bright side, sleeping for the recommended number of hours each night helps leave you feeling refreshed and ready to take on the day. This often helps motivate people to increase their amount of exercise. Not only does this positive habit help decrease the risk of weight gain, diabetes, and heart disease, it can also help you sleep more soundly at night.

Sleep Deprivation Mimics Prediabetes

Most people are familiar with diabetes. With an estimated 30 million people (10 percent of the population) in the United States diagnosed with some form of the disease, it's likely that everyone actually knows someone who has it. Moreover, there are an estimated seven million people that have diabetes and haven't been diagnosed yet. However, prior to getting type 2 diabetes, the most common form, people must go through a period of prediabetes. Sometimes known as insulin resistance, this stage can eventually lead to full-fledged diabetes if it is not controlled. Interestingly, chronic sleep deprivation can cause symptoms that mimic prediabetes. For example, a person is more likely to experience high blood sugar, resistance to insulin, and weight gain. The chronic negative effects of true diabetes are well-documented. As such, it's important to get control of the disease before it progresses from this intermediate state.

Studies have shown that those experiencing prediabetic symptoms due to chronic sleep loss often see them disappear once their sleep schedule is regulated. By helping regulate and maintain the body's metabolism, getting enough hours of high-quality sleep can be a helpful tool for fending off diabetes.

Not Sleeping Leads to Weight Gain

Like athletic recovery, the connection between sleep and metabolism revolves around hormones. When the body slows down at nighttime, it deploys a chemical soup of them to maintain its functions despite not getting any new fuel for several hours at a time. Interestingly enough, experts believe that the metabolic rate actually decreases by about 15 percent during sleep. While this might seem counterintuitive, the previously discussed factors like insulin sensitivity and leptin maintenance play a major role in reducing weight gain and regulating the daytime metabolism.

Like most things, the body does a tremendous job of adapting to short term disturbances in sleep. As such, it's not likely that only getting three hours of sleep for one night is going to contribute to weight gain. Unfortunately, during extended periods of sleep deprivation, like those experienced by a third of the population, the body is less adept at coping. With a decreased ability to process sugar, more cravings for unhealthy foods, and less motivation to exercise, those who don't get enough sleep are at a higher risk of gaining weight.

Fortunately, increasing your nightly sleep to the recommended level may actually help you lose some weight. Those already sleeping for seven hours a night probably won't see much of a difference on the scale by adding an extra half hour. However, a person that consistently gets five hours and ups that number to seven could see the scale start dropping. When it comes to regulating and maintaining the body, there's no better method than sleep. For those looking for help losing a few pounds, and those that just don't want to add any, the metabolic benefits of getting enough sleep are massive.

PART THREE

Mental Benefits of Sleep

CHAPTER 8

Sleep Improves Learning and Memory

With all of the physical benefits that sleep provides, it's easy to forget that there are plenty more which are a little harder to see. Although sleeping gives the body a chance to repair itself and recover, it is also crucial to the brain. From cleaning out toxins to forming memories, sleep is just as important for the mind as it is for the body. The psychological benefits of sleep are plentiful. By getting the recommended amount of sleep each night, individuals can see results like increased memory, easier learning, a boost in their mood, and even a decreased risk for mental health conditions like depression and anxiety.

As of now, research in the area of sleep and cognition is still developing. However, studies are beginning to show that there is indeed a correlation between the two. On the other hand, science has shown that being extremely sleep deprived is comparable to being intoxicated. For those in rigorous college majors, thought-provoking jobs, or anyone that feels like they could be better at remembering things, forming an ideal sleep routine is the first place to start. Not only are studies showing that sleep can increase problem solving skills and boost memory recall, they also show that people who are well-rested are able to learn better and be more productively than those who aren't. With those benefits in mind, let's examine why sleeping has such a large impact on cognition.

Sleep and Learning

One of sleep's most important cognitive functions is that of facilitating learning. Although it is commonly believed that learning happens during the day, a crucial part of the process occurs overnight while the learner is asleep. To better understand this, it's important to know that learning is divided into three stages—acquisition, consolidation, and recall. The first of these, acquisition, occurs when someone is introduced to new information. For example, when they first read a new fact from a textbook or hear it from a teacher. We'll come back to consolidation in a moment. The third step, recall, occurs when someone accesses that information once again at some point in the future. Both acquisition and recall can only consciously occur when a person is awake, which makes sense. You can't learn something new while you're sleeping. Nor can you knowingly conjure up a fun fact in the middle of a dream. However, brain patterns during sleep help facilitate the middle stage of learning: consolidation. This refers to the process carried out within the brain to stabilize and store a memory to prepare it for long-term recall. Though it is possible for consolidation to happen while someone is awake, it most frequently occurs during sleep. Research has not yet proven exactly how this occurs. However, it is believed that stage two of light sleep, along with REM, are the periods most associated with long-term memory consolidation.

Since consolidation plays a key role in helping people learn, the natural connection is that getting more sleep can help boost memory formation and future recall. It's worth noting that memory can be further divided into two categories: declarative (*what* you know) and procedural (*how* to do things). However, since research of sleep's impact on learning is still so convoluted, it's difficult to separate the two. Indeed, most research actually suggests that sleep improves learning and memory formation of both types. Regardless, getting more sleep will help facilitate the transfer of information into long-term storage within the brain. For those hoping to retain knowledge of new facts or techniques, getting more sleep is a valuable ally. This is also one instance where napping could be helpful. Although everyone should focus on getting at least seven hours of uninterrupted sleep at night, taking a brief nap during the daytime, especially after a study session, could help improve future recall. Since stage two sleep plays a role in memory consolidation, napping for around 90 minutes can allow the brain to "catch up" and store the recently learned information before it is lost to the events of the rest of the day.

Despite all of this, sleep doesn't just affect the consolidation process. It also plays an indirect role in the acquisition phase. A person who gets less sleep at night is more likely to wake up sleepy, grouchy, and "foggy." As a result, they will have difficulty with the acquisition stage of the learning process. Someone who is less vigilant due to a lack of sleep also won't be able to maintain their attention span as long as someone who is well rested. By contrast, a well-rested individual will be able to acquire new information far more effectively. So, while sleep deprivation affects the consolidation stage, it can also prevent memories from even getting there in the first place. This twofold effect is a great reason why those trying to learn new information should focus on getting enough sleep. Doing so helps you pay closer attention to new material, critically think through it, and eventually retain it as a long-term memory.

Sleep and Problem-Solving

Another critical cognitive component affected by sleep is problem-solving. Although most problems are solved during the day, research has shown that some, especially difficult problems, are better approached from a bed than a desk.

A Lancaster University study gave groups of individuals several tasks of varying difficulty to solve. After an initial attempt to solve the puzzle, each group was given a different path to follow. One group took a break and slept, eventually achieving REM sleep. Another also took a break but remained awake. The third group had no delay and was forced to continue trying to solve the problem. Interestingly, the group that was allowed to "sleep on" their problem solved more difficult puzzles than participants in the other groups. Researchers noted that there was no difference in the solving of easy puzzles, only difficult ones. It is believed that the discrepancy between the groups can be attributed to a concept known as spreading activation. While in REM sleep, the brain reactivates certain information related to the problem. This, in turn, activates the entire neural network related to solving the problem and gave participants an enhanced ability to solve the problem when they woke up. Along the same lines, a study from Harvard Medical School found that participants waking up from REM sleep were able to solve 30 percent more problems than those awoken from non-REM sleep. Again, the research showed that this boost relates to the solving of complex problems.

Sleep is the Best Teacher

Everyone has their own strategies for learning. Some find it easier than others. Though two people sit through the same lecture, they may recall entirely different portions of the information on an exam. A team of two engineers might approach a difficult problem in two totally unique ways. Learning is, after all, an individual activity. No one else can facilitate the acquisition, consolidation, and recall process. Yet, sleep is the common denominator that enhances learning for everyone. Whether a person is a visual learner, an audible learner, or prefers to learn by getting their hands dirty and doing something in person, sleep can improve the quality of the knowledge gained. It, for one, improves alertness and attention spans. Once a well-rested person first learns new information, getting the recommended amount of sleep that night then helps them consolidate it and store it in their long-term memory for a later date. When it's time to approach a tough problem, someone who takes time to sleep on it has a better chance of coming to a solution than someone that struggles through it without taking time to rest. Although sleeping can feel like a waste of time when studying and learning take place during the daytime, it should not be overlooked. Rather, those hoping to boost their cognition should prioritize getting enough sleep and close their eyes peacefully, knowing that sleeping will enhance learning and problem-solving more than any other strategy.

CHAPTER 9

Sleep Can Improve Your Mood

Everyone has been there at some point. The familiar sound of the alarm clock going off way too early. The bad mood that's sure to follow for the rest of the day. Whether it's a toddler throwing a temper tantrum after not getting a nap or an adult with road rage on the way home from a long day at work, not getting enough sleep can seriously impact your mood. Many people try to just "suck it up" and go about their business while pretending that their mood isn't affected. However, that isn't the best strategy for success. Science has shown that having a sleep debt is linked to anger, depression, and stress.

Fortunately, that doesn't have to be the case. By reversing a sleep debt, or by increasing the amount of sleep you currently get, you can actually boost your mood and feel happier going through the day. Something as simple as sleeping for the recommended seven to eight hours each night can greatly improve your happiness and quality of life. But why is sleep so connected to our moods?

An Angry Amygdala

Many people find it interesting to learn that the brain actually has a special section for regulating the emotions. No, it's not like Disney's "Inside Out" control center. Yet, the limbic system does serve as the primary influence over our emotions. Since emotions aren't a tangible or universally measured thing, research surrounding them is often inconclusive. Much remains unknown about why humans feel the things they feel when they feel them. However, there are a few features that are known to play a role in the regulation of our emotions. One of these is the amygdala. This almond-shaped portion of the brain is nestled near the hippocampus and the anterior portion of the temporal lobe. Actually, there are two amygdalae. One rests in either hemisphere of the brain. These tiny bundles of nerves help process stressful or frightening signals and mount a "fight or flight" response. The amygdala is also responsible for helping to process intense emotional reactions like fear and anger.

New research is beginning to uncover a previously unknown link between the amygdala and sleep deprivation. One study found that male participants who slept less had higher scores for anger on the Buss-Perry Aggression Questionnaire. Along the same lines, the study found that women are susceptible to having a depressed mood, anxiety, and brain fog when missing out on sleep. In children, both mood changes and behavior changes were noted. While these results do show a correlation between less sleep and a poor mood, researchers weren't able to narrow down the exact cause. That is, until another study from Japan's National Institute of Mental Health found that a sleep debt decreases the medial prefrontal cortex's ability to suppress the amygdala's activity. When the amygdala is left unchecked, it leads to mood swings and anger. While more studies are needed to confirm these findings, they are a likely indication that the amygdala is a primary culprit for the mood swings experienced by those that don't get enough sleep.

It Goes Both Ways

Have you ever tried to go to bed angry? If so, you probably didn't have much success—at least not at first. With thoughts rolling around in your mind, an elevated blood pressure, shallow breathing, and a faster heart rate, it's no wonder that being angry can disrupt sleep. Even though many people think of a lack of sleep as a cause of mood disturbances, it actually goes both ways. Going to bed either sad or in a bad mood can decrease the quality of sleep that you get and make the cycle worse the next day. Much of this has to do with the interactions between hormones in your brain. "Happy" hormones like serotonin and dopamine are believed to play a role in the creation of melatonin, which helps the body fall asleep. Understandably, when someone is in a bad mood and these levels are lower than when they are happy. At bedtime, this can mean there is less melatonin produced.

While not getting enough sleep certainly causes mood disturbances, it's important to remember that your mood going into bedtime has a lot to do with the quality of rest that you'll get that night. With that in mind, it's easy to see the importance of establishing a relaxing nighttime routine. By allowing your mind and body to calm down before bed, you can increase not only your sleep quality but your mood the next day. Sometimes it will be extremely difficult to get into a good mood before bed—especially if the day was taxing. However, at least attempting to do something that puts a smile on your face can give your happy hormones the boost that they need to help facilitate restful sleep. Many people find that a calm activity like reading a book helps them achieve a happier state before falling asleep. Others enjoy a warm shower or some relaxing music to boost their mood. In all reality, the activity you do to get happy before bed doesn't matter so long as it helps put you in a good mood. Establishing a routine that includes a mood-boosting activity before bed can help escape the cycle of bad moods leading to bad sleep and vice versa.

A Simple Solution

For those who don't get enough sleep, it might be hard to remember the last time they were in a great mood for an entire day without feeling worn out. Previously, we discussed the various physical problems that can occur due to a lack of sleep. Many of these, unfortunately, are difficult to reverse once they are allowed to get out of control. For example, reversing the prediabetes found in those who are chronically sleep deprived requires not only an adjusted sleep schedule but also various lifestyle modifications like dieting and exercise. On the other hand, our mood is highly adaptive and responds well when sleep problems are addressed. Those in a poor mood after a few nights of sleep debt will typically see their symptoms go away once they sleep well for about a week. Even people who are chronically sleep deprived can improve their mood. Though that process will certainly take longer, it is possible. Yet, it all relies on paying off your sleep debt. For some, it might take a few months on a healthy sleep schedule to fully rid themselves of a daily bad mood. For others, it will be a gradual improvement as they get their sleep habits on a better course.

Mood is just one more reason why getting the recommended seven to eight hours of nightly sleep is crucial. For many, it might be the first step in reversing the negative physical effects of chronic sleep loss. After all, those who wake up in a positive mood are more likely to embrace other healthy changes like diet and exercise. However, everyone can benefit from a mood boost—whether they have physical problems related to sleep loss or not. Waking up happier can lead to better relationships, self-esteem, and more creativity. Plus, who doesn't love feeling happy? Like many other things, sleep is at the core of our mood. Getting enough of it will help ensure that it remains positive.

CHAPTER 10

Poor Sleep is Linked to Depression and Anxiety

We've discussed the link between sleep and mood changes. While not getting enough hours of rest can leave someone in a bad mood the problem only gets worse over time. If a sleep disturbance is not controlled, it can quickly spiral into a full-blown sleep disorder like insomnia, hypersomnia, or narcolepsy. Studies show strong evidence that these conditions share a relationship with mental health conditions like depression and anxiety. Furthermore, such conditions on their own can lead to altered sleep patterns.

It's important to note that, once a sleep problem progresses to this state, reversing it by getting more hours in bed isn't the best course of action. Mental health disorders like depression and anxiety should be treated by a professional that is trained to do so. Treatments like therapy or psychological medications are often necessary to manage the disorder and sleep alone won't "fix" it. However, good sleep habits may help prevent them from developing in the first place.

Sleep and Depression Share a Close Relationship

Consistent data from countless studies has shown that depression and sleep are closely intertwined. Not only in the way that they affect each other once a person is diagnosed but also in regard to how often they are diagnosed concomitantly. The National Sleep Foundation's "Sleep in America" poll found that 18 percent of adults between the ages of 18 to 64 have been clinically diagnosed with depression. On top of this, these individuals were more likely to report a sleep disorder at the same time. Another poll of adolescents from the ages of 11 to 17 found that 73 percent who reported feeling unhappy also reported that they do not get the recommended amount of sleep each night. Finally, National Sleep Foundation data suggests that those who suffer from insomnia are 10 times more likely to develop depression and a whopping 17 times more likely to develop anxiety than someone who sleeps normally.

Feeling sad every once in a while is normal. In fact, it's healthy. No one can feel happy and enthusiastic all day every day when the trials of life get in the way. However, the persistent sadness and loss of interest in daily activities experienced by those with depression isn't something that most people experience. Interestingly, sleep disturbances are often the first signs of depression. Many clinical providers are able to diagnose a mental health condition based on the way a person's sleep is being affected. Unfortunately, this can also lead to many misdiagnoses of either a sleep disorder or mood disorder because the two share such similar symptoms. Nonetheless, sleep and depression are tightly, remarkably linked. Some have gone so far as to describe sleep disturbances as a classical sign of depression.

So, why does this relationship exist? A University of Chicago study showed that fundamental changes in sleep architecture, the way the body and brain function during sleep, are linked with depression. For one, the continuity of sleep is often disrupted. In other words, those with depression experience more periods of wakefulness during the night and those periods often last longer than those of someone without depression. Likewise, depressed individuals experienced less restorative slow wave sleep than those in a control group. Several alterations in REM sleep also occurred, some of which persisted even once a person's depression entered remission.

Sleep and Anxiety

Oftentimes when mental health issues are discussed, depression and anxiety appear side by side. That's not a coincidence. Not only do the two conditions share many characteristics, they also share many risk factors. Both depression and anxiety also feature a connection to sleep. Individuals suffering from anxiety often experience new or worsened sleep disruptions—much like those with depression. The mind-racing, heart pounding symptoms of anxiety can make it impossible to fall asleep at night. Then, seeing the clock tick onward towards the morning doubles the anxiety and makes it even harder to fall asleep.

Data from the National Institute of Mental Health found that between 24-36 percent of patients with a diagnosed anxiety disorder also had some degree of insomnia. A further 27-42 percent exhibited signs of hypersomnia (excessive sleepiness). Like depression, sleep disorders are a telling sign of an underlying mental health condition and doctors often rely on problems during sleep to diagnose the latter. Among the adult population, anxiety is the most common mental health condition. Considering that a third of adults also don't get the recommended amount of sleep each night, this fact isn't surprising. Rather, it serves to demonstrate the link between anxiety and a lack of sleep.

Managing Sleep Doesn't Treat Mental Health Conditions but it Can Help Prevent Them

Both anxiety and depression (as well as other mental health conditions) should be evaluated and treated by a professional. However, those who are currently not getting enough sleep should know that doing so puts them at an increased risk of developing a psychological disorder. Likewise, those struggling to fall asleep or stay asleep are also at higher risk. Though scientists have not yet determined every way in which sleep affects the brain, some key points have been identified. For one, sleep disturbances alter the levels of various hormones and neurotransmitters in the brain. When these levels are thrown off, the brain is no longer able to function at its peak. Over time, this can lead to the development of problems like anxiety and depression.

Though this all sounds pretty bleak, there is some hope. Since sleep and mental health conditions are so closely linked, ensuring that the quality of sleep is good can help prevent them from occurring. Some people are genetically predisposed to developing a disorder like depression or anxiety. For these individuals, getting proper sleep is even more important. Despite the increased risk, it could still help prevent a mental health disorder from occurring. According to Harvard Medical School, making positive lifestyle changes, establishing good sleep hygiene, and maintaining an aerobic exercise routine can all help improve the quality of sleep for those suffering from sleep disturbances. Doing so will not only improve your mood in the short term but also help limit the risk of mental health disorders. Part four of this book will explore different ways to establish good sleep habits. Meanwhile, people who aren't experiencing problems sleeping but still don't get enough hours in bed should make paying off their sleep debt a priority. Although sleep alone isn't going to cure depression or anxiety, it is still something very important to consider—especially as it relates to prevention.

Sleep in Action

With the many health benefits, both mental and physical, of sleep in mind, you might be wondering how you can start achieving them in your own life. As mentioned several times throughout the course of this book, sleep routines are different for everyone. What works for you might not work for a co-worker. The way you prepare for sleep will be different than how your child gets ready for bed. Keeping this in mind is a very important part of putting sleep into action. By allowing yourself to embrace the sleep routine that is perfect for you, each night will become more restful and more beneficial to your health.

One of the best ways to enhance your quality of sleep is to establish a good sleep hygiene routine. No, this doesn't mean taking a shower before bed. Sleep hygiene refers to a set of activities that you practice throughout the day which affect your quality of rest at night. For example, not having caffeine or nicotine within a few hours of bedtime can help your body stay asleep throughout the entire night rather than experiencing disruptions in the latter half. These lifestyle habits bolster the quality of sleep you get each night and affect how you are able to unlock the benefits of sleeping.

Creating a healthy sleep hygiene routine is easier than it sounds. Most of these activities will take place near or right before bedtime. However, some, like napping, can occur throughout the day. Although a nap during the day can be refreshing and help make you feel more alert, it can also disrupt your nighttime sleep. So, you should avoid taking regular naps longer than 30 minutes to keep your sleep cycle intact. Another daytime sleep hygiene practice is to create an exercise routine. The National Sleep Foundation states that as little as 10 minutes of daily aerobic exercise can improve your sleep quality at night. With that being said, it's important to not exercise too close to bedtime as that can have the opposite effect. When it starts getting late, there are some other activities to keep in mind. For one, you should try to limit your exposure to natural light and other bright lights. These can disrupt your body's natural sleep-wake cycle and make it harder to fall asleep. Though it will come as sad news to some, the light emitted by devices like smartphones and televisions has the same effect. As such, you should aim to turn off your technology at least an hour before you plan to go to sleep.

On top of this, creating a bedtime routine or ritual is a key part of good sleep hygiene. Over time, this trains your body to start relaxing and get ready for bed. You should ideally repeat the same routine every night. Many people like to start with a warm shower or bath to clear their mind and begin the relaxation process. Then, try brushing your teeth, washing your face, and taking out your contacts if you wear them. Once you climb into bed, you should feel calm, clean, and ready to get some rest. Even once you get there, you can still take time to unwind before falling asleep. A calm activity like reading a book, meditating, or even just listening to calming music can put your body in a state of relaxation. By repeating this routine every night, your body will start to establish it as a regular part of your sleep cycle. Not only does this make it easier to fall asleep once you're ready, it can improve the quality of sleep you get.

There are so many benefits to getting good sleep. From a healthier immune system to a healthier heart and quicker metabolism, the sleep you get each night affects your body in many ways. Getting enough of it can leave you feeling happier, healthier, and more like yourself. On the contrary, being sleep deprived makes you moody and puts you at a higher risk for mental health conditions like depression and anxiety. For athletes, desk jockeys, students, children, the elderly, and everyone in between, sleep is a crucial part of your health. Though many people see it as something that can be overlooked, the truth is, you can't afford to. With all of the good things that sleep has to offer, there has never been more incentive to lay down, close your eyes, and drift off into better health.

References

Chapter 1:

http://www.ncbi.nlm.nih.gov/pubmed/12683469

https://academic.oup.com/sleep/article/42/2/
zsy221/5185637

https://www.cdc.gov/sleep/about_sleep/how_much_
sleep.html

https://www.sleepfoundation.org/articles/teens-and-sleep

https://www.sleepfoundation.org/articles/aging-and-sleep

Chapter 2:

https://www.ncbi.nlm.nih.gov/books/NBK19961/

https://www.ncbi.nlm.nih.gov/books/NBK19961/

https://www.mayoclinic.org/diseases-conditions/high-blood-pressure/expert-answers/sleep-deprivation/faq-20057959

Chapter 3:

https://www.ninds.nih.gov/Disorders/Patient-Caregiver-Education/Understanding-Sleep

https://www.sleep.org/articles/what-happens-during-sleep/

Chapter 4:

https://www.ncbi.nlm.nih.gov/pmc/articles/PMC3256323/

https://journals.sagepub.com/doi/full/10.1111/j.1467-8721.2007.00468.x

https://www.tchc.org/blog/2018/12/12/hand-hygiene-and-germ-facts/

https://www.cdc.gov/handwashing/why-handwashing.html

Chapter 5:

https://www.ncbi.nlm.nih.gov/pubmed/10234087

https://www.sleepfoundation.org/excessive-sleepiness/health-impact/how-sleep-deprivation-affects-your-heart

Chapter 6:

https://www.wm.edu/offices/
sportsmedicine/_documents/sleep-manual

Chapter 7:

https://www.niddk.nih.gov/health-information/
health-statistics/overweight-obesity

https://www.ncbi.nlm.nih.gov/pubmed/15531540

https://www.diabetesresearch.org/diabetes-statistics

Chapter 8:

https://www.ncbi.nlm.nih.gov/pubmed/19379769

http://healthysleep.med.harvard.edu/healthy/matters/
benefits-of-sleep/learning-memory

https://doi.org/10.3758/s13421-012-0256-7

http://www.pnas.org/content/99/26/16519.full

Chapter 9:

https://www.ncbi.nlm.nih.gov/pubmed/24693810/

https://www.ncbi.nlm.nih.gov/pubmed/28977527

http://healthysleep.med.harvard.edu/need-sleep/
whats-in-it-for-you/mood

Chapter 10:

https://www.sleepfoundation.org/articles/
depression-and-sleep

https://www.ncbi.nlm.nih.gov/pmc/articles/
PMC3181883/

https://www.health.harvard.edu/newsletter_article/
sleep-and-mental-health

Part 4:

https://www.sleepfoundation.org/articles/sleep-hygiene

About the Authors

reg Justice is a best-selling author, speaker, and fitness entrepreneur and was inducted into the National Fitness Hall of Fame in 2017. He founded **AYC Health & Fitness**, Kansas City's Original Personal Training Center, in May 1986. Greg co-founded **Scriptor Publishing Group** and the **National Corporate Fitness Institute** (NCFI), a certifying body for fitness professionals.

He has been actively involved in the fitness industry for four decades as a club manager, owner, personal fitness trainer, and corporate wellness supervisor. He has worked with athletes and non-athletes of all ages and physical abilities and served as a conditioning coach at the collegiate level. He worked with the Kansas City Chiefs, during the offseason, in the early 1980's, along with professional baseball, soccer and golf athletes.

Greg has authored or co-authored 25+ books including, *Treadside Manner: Confessions of a Serial Personal Trainer* and *Mind Your Own Fitness: A Mindful Approach to Exercise*, and contributes to many international publications including, Men's Fitness, Women's Health, Prevention, Time, US News & World Report, New York Times, IDEA Fitness Journal, Corporate Wellness Magazine, and writes a monthly column for Personal Fitness Professional magazine.

Greg holds a master's degree in HPER (exercise science) (1986) and a bachelor's degree in Health & Physical Education (1983) from Morehead State University, Morehead, KY. He also holds many industry certifications.

Greg is available for speaking engagements. You may contact Greg at info@GregJustice.com, or visit www.GregJustice.com for more information.

Art Still is a writer, speaker and CEO of Still 4 Life, an ecommerce business that believes in "paying it forward".

He was born and raised in Camden, New Jersey where he graduated from Camden High School in 1974.

Art was a four year starter at the University of Kentucky, where he was named SEC Player of the Year and Consensus All-American as a senior. He was inducted into the College Football Hall of Fame in 2015.

In 1978, Art was the first round draft pick of the Kansas City Chiefs and played 12 seasons in the NFL with the Chiefs and Buffalo Bills. He was selected to four Pro-Bowls, was a two time MVP, and inducted into the Kansas City Chiefs Hall of Fame in 1997.

In addition to a very active family life, Art has taken on various projects since he left the game, including charity work with several organizations. Still remains connected with football serving as one of the Chiefs ambassadors. In that role he is frequently out and about in the community with other former players. "You get an opportunity to work in the community with a variety of charities and groups of people," said Still, who has been married to wife Liz since

1982. "We enjoy doing things that are positive and something that will be lasting in helping others. We do a lot of benefits and working with youths and their families."

Art is available for speaking engagements. You may contact Art at support@Still4Life.com or visit www.Still4Life.com for more information.